To Lyna
Faithful
Faithful
Faithful
Much Love
Sista
Hooper

Egregious

Regina Lee Hooper

Egregious

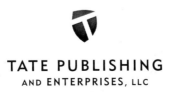

TATE PUBLISHING
AND ENTERPRISES, LLC

Published by Tate Publishing & Enterprises, LLC
127 E. Trade Center Terrace | Mustang, Oklahoma 73064 USA
1.888.361.9473 | www.tatepublishing.com

Tate Publishing is committed to excellence in the publishing industry. The company reflects the philosophy established by the founders, based on Psalm 68:11,
"The Lord gave the word and great was the company of those who published it."

Published in the United States of America

ISBN: 978-1-68118-066-3
1. Religion / Christian Ministry / Preaching
2. Health & Fitness / General
15.08.11

I dedicate this book to my mother,
Ann Lee.

To my husband, Thomas,
and to my Church family.

And above all, to Jesus Christ,
the author and creator of all living
beings in heaven and earth.

CONTENTS

PREFACE

I write this book from an urgent need to inform Americans of the health hazards that are standing at our door and the fundamental decisions that have been made on our behalf that have made many of us sick and if never corrected will continue to sicken us, if not kill many of us in great numbers.

Although this book may be small, I am reminded of a quote by Edwin Burke, statesmen, author, and philosopher: "It is a mistake to do nothing because one could only do little."

The information listed in this book is common knowledge, well-known, but never has any of it been given the constant front-page knowledge needed to change policies that control our health. All subjects listed below are some causes of why our lives are controlled the way they are.

After World War ll, Nuremberg, Germany, held several trials, most important to this discussion were the IG Farben trials (a massive pharmaceutical conglomerate that funded the war and enlarged the wealth of many robber baron dynasties). These three IG Farben defendants all indicted for crimes against humanity, terror, torture, slave labor, and more spent little time in jail and lived out their natural lives as free men:

Fritz ter Meer—chemist and supervisor, became chairman of a global pharmaceutical company;

Otto Ambrose—chemist and maker of nerve gases that killed millions, became a chemical advisor;

Max Bruggeman—indicted and excused because he was sick.

In the book *Emerging Viruses,* Dr. Leonard Horowitz gives and explanation of disease origins and "Operation Paperclip" (and much more) that allowed thousands of highly educated war criminals to enter America with identity changes to melt into the fabric of our society.

I pray to Jesus Christ, who knows all things, to give us grace and mercy to be saved from the hands of evil and give a season of peace on this earth and the right to freedom of health.

THE ORIGIN OF MAN

The theory of race is one that has caused and is causing wars, genocide, murders, and a great sense of unrest. The truth of all mankind is that Adam and Eve, who originated somewhere in Sub-Saharan Africa, were black-skinned people. Originally, all people all over the earth were black. Black people come in all tones—blue, black, caramel, beige, white, and tan. Africans have one of the highest rates of giving birth to children who have genes lacking sufficient hair, eye, and skin color; this is known as albinism.

Albinos producing offspring with darker-skinned people produce offspring mulatto in color. Very light-skinned black people constantly interbreeding produce a constant seeming race of light-skinned people, we have before called white. These people I will call our ancestral children. To offer the hatred that was directed at dark blacks at them will never do; we are all one race of people. We are all distant relatives of one black man and woman. The killing and the hatred must stop, especially the race-baiting done by America's television, radio, and print media. Acts 17:26 (King James Version) says that God has made of one blood all nations of mankind to live on the earth.

Among the ancestral children, there are issues the media completely hides or ignores or lies about. There are two million cases of head lice in North America annually. The Department of Health acknowledges that at any given time, 30 percent of school children of any color, mostly with clean, silky hair, will be infested with head lice. Instead of a routine monitoring of this issue, schools wait until there are living and active lice in the students' head; only then are they sent home to treat this condition. A regular routine of head checks and treating nits with intensity would avoid the embarrassment and singling out of students. This is ignored, and the public is bombarded with commercials of the beauty of silky hair.

On the other hand, in Africa, where there are less silky haired people and more curly, woolly haired people, the lice have adapted with claws on their legs, and there they afflict more woolly haired persons, who happen to usually be dark skinned. In order to have true peace, these issues have to be addressed as a fact of everyday life, and no shame should be attached to the issue, as each individual human makes a decision to live in peace. What identifies us as "races" of people—our hair, eye, and skin color—comprises less than 0.01 percent of gene expressions, so 99.99 percent of human beings are similar. We humans are unlike the animals. Their flesh are usually full of dangerous viruses harmful to humans.

The absolute truth of racism is that we are one race of people in different colors. That Caucasian are the albino offspring of black people that were able to survive in the cooler climate of Europe. These facts are discussed well by Dr. Ivan van Sertima (1935–2009, anthropologist, expert scholar in African studies) in his books and speeches (i.e., "Black Women in Antiquity" and *They Came Before Columbus*.)

Racial hatred based on the truth that a Caucasian family intermarrying and breeding children with people of color will be difficult to identify a "Caucasian" skin tone in three generations.

This is the reason for the murderous race hatred in our country. For this lie, murder, assassination, and martyrdom have occurred. In Selma, Alabama, the day after the march across the Edmund Pettus Bridge, many people of all colors silently lost their lives, never to be mourned by media for very long. The Lee family reunion of Selma, Alabama, took a bus tour along the route of the Selma-Montgomery March. Unbeknown to me, my mother had requested that we honor one of those brave people. On July 4, 2015, my family laid flowers at the grave of Detroit housewife Viola Grubb Liuzzo, whose life was martyred for her participation and support of the Selma march. Ms. Liuzzo was a person who saw human beings, not race. My hope is that her legacy would be a catalyst for change in our nation especially in these trying times.

The original ancient Egyptians were not suntanned but black-colored people who had the advanced knowledge of science, math, language, and electricity. Nikola Tesla, a Serbian-American inventor and genius, copied an unadorned pyramid that was thought in error to be a burial chamber and produced in Wardenclyffe in New York electricity in the early 1900s as the Egyptians had done centuries ago. Tesla wished to give free wireless electricity and communication to all mankind, but J. P. Morgan stopped the money flow as he could not put a meter on it, but now we have wireless communications, e-mail, and WiFi power, and we pay a lot of money to keep it going. I believe it is needed to continue the lie of the pyramids to feed evolutionary thoughts of the ignorance and helplessness of early man.

Jesus Christ was a black-skinned man. The original children of Israel were and still are dark-skinned people. Original paintings of biblical Christ's twelve disciples including Peter, the first pope was black. Europe once had dark-skinned kings and queens. As the monarchies filled with our ancestral children, they did not want to be known as dark. With the Renaissance, European popes and monarchs commissioned biblical paintings and recolored paintings of ancient kings and queens that literature called dark complexion or swarthy—meaning, dark-skinned.

The ancestral children have changed the names of and colors of quite famous people to take glory for what was never theirs alone but belonged to all of us. In the book *100 Amazing Facts About the Negro* by J. A. Rogers, fact number 8 gives a description of Beethoven by his intimate friend Frau Fischer as "short, stocky, broad shoulders, short neck, round nose, and blackish-brown complexion." Beethoven's friend and mentor, composer Joseph Haydn, is described as a blackamoor by Prince Paul Esterházy, who had been enchanted by the composer's music and wish to meet him face to face.

Alexander Dumas, author of *The Three Musketeers* and *The Count of Monte Cristo*, was described as a black Haitian mulatto. In further explanation of the Dumas's family history is the 2013 Pulitzer Prize–winning book called *The Black Count : Glory, Revolution, Betrayal, and the Real Count of Monte Cristo* by Tom Reiss. Few persons know that the twentieth Roman emperor was Septimius Severus, a dark-skinned man with negroid features. The reading of J. A. Rogers's book would be an enlightening experience for us all.

Instead we are fed with the idea that dark-skinned people are only slaves, which is untrue.

The European were disturbed by the intermarrying of light- and dark-skinned people, and it led to the first Holocaust, the genocide of the Herero people on Shark Island. The theory of evolution by Sir Charles Darwin and the use of the divine right of kings, which stated that no one should question them but God, were used as tools to give European royalty the right to conquer what they dictated to be savages. Even today, an international arrest warrant by a common law court called the ITCCS (International Tribunal into Crimes Church and State) for the involvement of extremely high-ranking European officials in stealing the land and wealth of the Canadian Indians and the routine murder and genocide of fifty thousand Indian children in residential schools. We must speak on behalf of the missing. America itself has many missing persons of every color. We must speak now before there is no one left to speak on our behalf, as we are reminded by the poem called "First They Came" by Pastor Martin Niemoller.

In the book *Medicinal Cannibalism in Early Modern English Literature and Culture* by Louise Noble, Europeans of all classes practiced the strange phenomenon of eating human flesh and drinking human blood as a form of medicine well into the nineteenth century. The use of human fat as facial cream was nothing unusual. In the 1970s, German geneticist Dr. Alex Van Der Eb produced vaccine components from the kidney of a human embryo now known as HEK293.

There is a longstanding issue with the fact that human embryo tissue is used to produce flavoring for soda, food, multiple vaccines, and antiaging creams.

The pro-life organization Children of God for Life have identified a disturbing number of mandatory vaccines that are grown in aborted fetal tissue. Vaccines to treat adenovirus, smallpox, even the developing Ebola virus, contain different aborted fetal cells such as WI-38, MRC-5, PERC6, RA273, and WI26 VA4-RDNA. The organization encourages the alternate use of vaccines grown in rabbit, hen, hamster, and monkey tissue. I would surely hope that all vaccines will be carefully reevaluated as we learn more of the different viruses that already live in monkey tissue, which I will discuss later. Humanity must consider 1 Corinthians 15:39 (New International Version Bible): "Not all flesh is the same. People have one kind of flesh, animals have another, birds another and fish another." Evolution attempts to say we are one flesh with animals. Science and the God who made us have exposed this as dangerously untrue.

Very little of what truly goes on in the world is told to us. We are lied to a lot by media in America. The truth is obstructed from our view by television, radio, and printed media, but may God hold the hands of those who withhold truth and produce blatant lies fully accountable.

THE ORIGIN OF BANKING

America has been under a criminal central bank called the Federal Reserve for a little over one hundred years. In 1913, the Federal Reserve Act was cooked up by a group of Jewish Bankers headed by the Rothschild/ Rockefeller desire to own our country's wealth. This act is a work of *treason* because it oversteps the constitution article 1 section 8, which gives Congress "the power to coin money and regulate the trade thereof." The feds print worthless paper tender and charge American interest to do it, spiraling us into a eighteen-trillion-dollar debt for money we could print ourselves. The Federal Reserve Bank can be found as the cause of most of our current problems. They have never been audited, and with the push of a button, they can switch us into deep poverty.

Alan Greenspan's increase of interest rates plunged our nation into a foreclosure crisis that continues to this day. Before 1975, New York state's residents went to college for *free*; our taxes paid for it.

After the New York Federal Bank rescued NYC from financial problems, college students have been paying increasing student loans, sending them into a deep debt before they got their first job.

The Federal Reserve Act gave the Federal Reserve the power over Fort Knox, where our gold is stored. No American politician can truly say anyone knows what is now in Fort Knox. Ben Bernake once boldly sat before a senate hearing and refused to explain what the Federal Reserve had done with billions of tax payer dollars.

The corruption around the Federal Reserve, or the central banks as they are called, can be found connected to several presidents who attempted to remove them.

President Abraham Lincoln was encouraged to fund the Civil War through a group of central banks. He refused, for he feared that would leave our country in deep debt; therefore, he observed the Constitution and ignored the central bankers and had Congress print greenbacks. He was assassinated.

In spring of 1963, President John F. Kennedy found out about the problem of the Federal Reserve and stopped their power. President Kennedy then allowed Congress to print Kennedy silver dollars for this reason and other issues rarely spoken. Our beloved president was assassinated in November 1963.

President Lyndon B. Johnson returned the power to print money to the Federal Reserve, increasing the national debt.

President Ronald Reagan called together an investigation called the Grace Commission. Its job was to find out where the American people's money was going. Peter Grace, a businessman, gave the report that not one penny of taxes collected through the Internal Revenue Service (IRS) goes to pay for anything on USA soil. When President Reagan spoke against the Federal Reserve and the IRS, an assassination attempt was made on his life. Thank God he survived, but he never spoke a bad word about the IRS, the Grace Commission findings, or the Federal Reserve.

Although we may not agree with everything a president does or says, we are cautioned by God's word to pray for them that they may be safe and they may be good examples to our nation.

As you read these words, the Federal Reserve now has control of America's money. The Federal Reserve now coins and regulates our money and is now in control of the SEC (Securities and Exchange Commission). Our system of checks and balance to keep any one part of our government from holding too much power has been breeched.

Thoma Jefferson, the third president of the United States, warned us if we allowed a central bank to coin and regulate our money, the corporations and banks that grow up around them would make us homeless on the land our fathers conquered. Abraham Lincoln once said that banks should only produce the money into circulation that is needed to run the country.

In Nehemiah chapter 5 (KJV) is found the answer to our dilemma—the abolishment of usury (egregiously high interest rates benefiting the lender) and the restoration and return of houses, lands, and property to their rightful owners.

VACCINATIONS

Jenner, the Father of Vaccines and Plagues

Sir Edward Jenner was a country doctor who was taught on a one-to-one basis by another country doctor. He brought his first credential for what would be seventy-five dollars today and begged the Royal Academy for entrance but when told that he would have to be tested, he declined, but was later admitted for a study of the cuckoo bird. He stole the idea of inoculation against small pox from a local farmer with pus from a cow—in Latin, *vacca*, hence the term *vaccination*.

The problem with smallpox is that it was a disease of poor sanitation and malnutrition, having ignored this fact. Many later university-taught physicians of his day came to see vaccination as the producer of disease as records began to prove that the already vaccinated caught disease and usually died first.

The little town of Leicester, England, adhered to strict sanitation and isolation for its sick and held the lowest rates of smallpox in England. Jenner's first patient, John Phipps, and his own son and wife all died of tuberculosis, long thought to be a result of seeding the human body with cow pus to make one healthy

Dr. Charles Creighton, a university-taught medical doctor and medical manuscript writer, wrote a thorough and balanced explanation of vaccination for Encyclopedia Britannica, which promptly disappeared after the books were brought by the Rockefeller Foundation and replaced with a report more favorable to vaccination. Wealthy philanthropists who routinely went to third-world nations give them "life-saving vaccines" that plunged the nation in debt while its citizens still suffered hunger, malnutrition, inadequate clothes, and no clean source of drinking water, the man's basic need. Dr. Jonas Salk (a medical doctor and noted virologist who created the first supposedly inactivated polio vaccine) went to his grave knowing that he had made a vaccine grown in the filthy kidney of monkeys that may well be the cause of spreading SV40, or simian virus 40, which produced latent cancers in laboratory animals. When Dr. Bernice Eddy began to understand that these same late-in-life cancers would show in the American population, she was demoted and quieted. In the book *The Virus and the Vaccine* by D. Bookchin and J. Schumacher, note that SV40 produces a mesothelioma-like cancer in persons never exposed to asbestos. American televisions are filled with law firms seeking plaintiffs to collect an 30-billion-dollar government trust for persons affected by mesothelioma. This throughly researched book also goes on to note that SV40 is a stealth virus and is transferable between human beings. Today one in three or one in four Americans are experiencing cancer and the alphabet agencies of our government knew this from the beginning. The pharmaceutical industry was so concerned about vaccine effectiveness that they were happy if only 10 percent of the population was helped by vaccines, the profits were enormous.

In the book *Dissolving Illusions* by Suzanne Humphries and Roman Bystrianyk in a thoroughly researched and informative description of the history of vaccines and disease, it is explained that large portions of the world population already have the measles and polio viruses in their body and never become sick until their immune system becomes disarmed through malnutrition, poor diet, and stress. The book goes on to explain the role nutrition, health, and misleading public health reports play in disease. I believe there is a much-needed area of research of our city's rising Hepatitis B. Is it possible it is due to the last twenty or more years of seeding the most innocent form of human life with a vaccine that would otherwise only be given to drug users who could spread this disease through needles, toiletries, sexual contact, and childbirth. But why not seek to test the mothers? Please consider the great possibility that vaccination is the cause of the increased disease rates; that and human behavior that sanctions the use of feces as normal.

Also explained in Dr. Humphries's book is America's lost Herbal Naturopathic and Homeopathic legacy. We are directed toward a hefty four-volume book called *Divided Legacy* by Harris L. Coulter. In portions of the book, you will come to understand how impatience, time itself, organized government groups, and the Flexner Report (Flexner Report was an evaluation of medical school in early twentieth century funded by the money of Robber Baron foundations that refused to fund most naturopathic based schools and greatly empowered medical schools that taught Allopathic medicine (medical teachings of surgery, synthetic prescription drugs, radiation, etc.). Benjamin Franklin once said, "Any nation that will give up its liberty for safety will eventually lose both." We must consider that when considering the possibility of a nationwide vaccination program and the removal of religious exemptions.

PASTEUR

The Crumbling Germ Theory

It was well-known for over a century that the germ theory on which vaccination rests is a shaky one. In textbooks, we are told that bacteria, fungi, and viruses are all different.

What came first was not germs but rundown immune systems and bodies due to lack of clean water and nutritious food and rest. A germ is a cell that changes shapes.

Louis Pasteur was a chemist, a microbiologist, a scoundrel, and a crook. It is long known that he stole the work of Pierre Jacques Antoine Béchamp, a gentleman, doctor, chemist, biologist, and professor. Pasteur made up the germ theory to feed the hungry mouths of pharmaceutical vaccinations. Dr. Bechamps coined and discovered microzyma, a living organism in human cells that morph when the body becomes weak, malnourished, and toxins appear. Microzyma begin to digest debris. Pasteur stole the word and changed it to microbe and called it the cause of disease. (Today Dr. Gaston Naessens has many studies into polymorphism of cells he calls somatids and has built a microscope called the somatiscope that may well change medicine forever.)

So disreputable were Pasteur studies and lab work that on his deathbed, he requested his papers never be opened to public view. After the death of his last close relative, his papers were opened to public view, and it has been on books and articles that Pasteur did steal the work of his colleagues and bullied them into silence with his overbearing presence and political clout. The United States government holds a patent on a strain of Ebola and as no one, not even the

US surgeon general, speaks any words of warning or proper common sense, we may as well expect our government to mandate compulsory vaccination for American citizens followed by mass deaths and a big profits for vaccine makers.

Today we stand at the door of mandated vaccines for people of every age. In the early 1900s, a young girl named Marcella Gruelle died of the side effects of a mandated smallpox vaccine that had been given several times at school. Her parents had no choice. The story goes on that her father, Johnny Gruelle, a political cartoonist and the creator of the Raggedy Ann and Andy doll and stories protested. Raggedy

Ann at one time was a symbol of the anti-vaccination movement in America.

As we speak, there are two kinds of consent in New York City schools. Informed consent must be signed by parent or guardian, or your child will miss school trips. However, passive consent is also used. Notes are sent home with the children. The parent may or may not receive the paper, but if there is no response, the program involving the student will go on. Usually the programs are very helpful, such as nutritional counseling or training in better asthma management to prevent unneeded absences and death from asthma. This passive consent is also being used to give free birth control and a morning-after abortion pill. It is called the

CATCH program (Connecting Adolescents to Comprehensive Health), given to girls as young as twelve. New York City has lowered the age of sexual consent to twelve years old, and most hardworking parents do not have a clue. This and artful public nakedness in NYC due to a little-known court decision from "The People and C., Respondent v. Romona Santorelli and Mary Lou Schloss," decided July 7, 1992.

This needs to be stopped. Parents, educators, and politicians must speak up.

In regard to the side effects of vaccine, there is one that parents are quite clueless about. In the treatment of anaphylaxis in American schools, there is a very necessary multibillion-dollar business of injectable, epinephrine. The origin of anaphylaxis is an interesting one, an explanation researched by Heather Frasier in her book *The Peanut Allergy Epidemic.* Dr. Charles Richet (1850–1935, French immunologist) won a Nobel Peace Prize for his study and coining of the word *anaphylaxis,* which means "against protection." Vaccination violates the human body's digestive system's ability to protect itself from the invasion of foreign proteins. He injected dogs with a protein that sensitized them and then injected them a second time. This caused anaphylaxis, and all the dogs died. Richet was a eugenicist (a person who believes in the removal of weak, sick, and inferior races of humans to improve the human gene pool). At one point in our history, peanut oil was added to vaccines as an adjuvant (antibody and immune system stimulant), and when children began to fall ill and simply drop dead, the scientific response was to build a multibillion-dollar industry to "save" them instead of admitting that vaccines were the cause. American courts removed the pharmaceutical companies accountability for the injury and death of human beings. A small portion of money is set aside from each vaccine sold to pay for vaccine-injured children and adults in a special court. To date, millions have been paid out. Are we chattel, or are we humans?

HEALTH IN AMERICA

Fluoridation

Fluoride is a halogen chemical, which means it mixes easily with other chemicals.

Fluoride is present in the United States drinking, cooking, and bathing water. There is no regulation of the dose from infant to adult. The medicating of water is against my constitutional right to be secure in my own person. Fluoride is a sedative; for example, valium plus fluoride equals rophies, the date rape drug that renders victims unconscious. Hitler added fluoride to the drinking water of concentration camp prisoners to make them more docile and easier to manage. We are being drugged.

Fluoride also causes ADHD and the slowing down of nervous system. Pharmaceutical companies are on the verge of medicating hundreds of school-age children on low-dose amphetamines, which are only gateway drugs to cocaine and other hard drugs, just as marijuana is a gateway drug to harder drug use.

The Prayer

Please keep our country safe from the threat of increasing disease that plague us. Please allow vaccination to be known for the harm it truly is.

If my people which are called by my name will humble themselves and pray and seek my face, then will I

hear from heaven and heal
their land.

—2 Chronicles 7:14 (KJV)

We pray that the central banks and the Federal Reserve will not destroy our nation; that every stolen and diverted portion of our nation's wealth will be returned; that every politician, every supreme court justice that is being bribed and/or extorting will be exposed and removed for failure to uphold our Constitutional Republic from harm for refusing to uphold the will of the people; that any politician imprisoned and scandalized maliciously or wrongfully will be released, and those at the foundation of their harm will be removed from places of power, wherever they be. We pray for corporations   and robber baron dynasties, former presidents and persons with power who have subverted the laws of our nation that they will be brought to their knees and removed; that a government by the people, for the people, and of the people will rise again; that this nation will have seated in government persons who will represent the will of God for this great nation; and that we shall not fall but rise again to be restored to a greater place of glory. We decree and declare divine order to every aspect of American life that has fallen into disorder. We decree and declare help, open doors, completion and closure for the work of "The International Tribunal for Crimes of Church and State" and healing for all disenfranchised persons all over the world. Please deliver us from the insanity of these plans for our destruction. In the name of Jesus Christ, amen.

"When Should I Mind My Business?"

by

Regina Lee Hooper

First define "my business"

Then define exactly

What is to

Quote ,unquote

"to mind"

I have heard before from another source

"It takes six months to mind
my own business"
"And six months to leave everyone
elses business alone"
Is homelesness my business?
Is the unfeed hungry child the
one in five my business?
Is the job offered but not taken my business?
Is the one on welfare because they would
make less working my business?
Are the brain injured my business?
Are the crys, spasms and destruction of
the human genome my business?
Are quiet genocides my business?
Science so precise , they can bypass bloody
sidewalks and broken buildings
and go straight for their target.

Our nerves, our lungs, our liver.
Are toxins my business?
Is the chemical bath I live in
daily my business?
When chemical sweetener
components and toxic additives
wind up in my hair treatment
bypassing my mouth and settling straight
into my follicles, my blood stream,
open access to my whole body
is that my business?
Where does it stop?
And exactly how much of my
business do I mind?

"POISONED WATERS"

by

Regina Lee Hooper

A lot of trouble

A gross of knowledge

To make poison sweet

To make harm subtle

To make harm caring

To make water clear

Effervescent to a sparkle

Descendants of the Manhattan Project

Requests a testing

Not of water, of other things

Mullenix knew, knew all too well

The mice were sick

The mice were slow

They did not learn

They did not know

Phyllis knew and she knew the name

She must go

Silence please the professional thought.

Was it known

Known of days gone by.

About Waldbott's "The Great Dilemma"

The softer bones

The cancers grow

No harm, no harm

More mice to catch

In sticky webs

Human mice

The pills will flow

Suicides so slow

Psychotic breaks

The white lights flash

The people die

The mice were sick

The mice were slow

They could not learn

They did not know

The guns will go

And the pills will flow

The mice were sick

And more will die

They did not know

They did not know

Now that you know, do something!

(Please research the work of

Dr. Phyllis Mullenix, PhD.)

"WHO LIED ABOUT THE TREES?"

by

Regina Lee Hooper

Deep in the quiet of the forest green

As furry little creatures run to and fro

I heard it! I heard it!

They said filing was obsolete

We could cut down on manpower

Less secretaries, less filing clerks

Less people

People are so expensive

Less jobs

Who said I was antiquated.

I have found myself

to be very reliable

Down thorough the years.

Under lock and key

Your secrets were safe always safe with me.

You just had to be careful who

you gave the key to.

To delete or alter precious words

stored on my pages

You had to cross me out

You had to abridge me

You had to send me back to production

Now with the silent stroke

The touch of a human finger

Truths long known are gone as

though they never existed.

The tree said "I miss the human touch"

Children used to adore me,

their stubby little fingers eagerly

writing on my soft pages.

I watched their print turn into script

I saw their progress

Now they ignore me

for little plastic boxes with lights,

batteries and mind altering

sequences

I used to be held warmly with affection

In the folds of their arms as they walked

To and from school

I heard their whispers to close friends

I felt the drops of their tears

When they were betrayed by all too young love

I was their first journal

I kept their innermost secrets

I never told a soul

Until someone, usually someone close

stole the key and read the words

Internet chat lines, fooled you

Fooled you big time

I would laugh if it wasn't such a pitiful mess

Put your innermost thoughts,

secrets and feelings

To only God knows who

On the World Wide Web

If privacy is a concept never learned

It cannot be missed when stolen away

People from one end of the earth to

the other can read your stuff

Come Precious tell me

Tell silver all about it

Tell me what you are thinking

Tell me where you've been

Tell me how you be

The silver rings never lie

tell me for posterity's sake

Write, write ,please write it on line

I only promise to tell your boss,

the social worker from ACS

And the people by the water cooler when

Jerry hacks the depths of my silver little soul

Oh yeah and I told the lady from Human

Resources at the job you wanted so badly.

That you were often depressed

and occasionally you drank too much

I showed her your Mardi Gras pictures

Yes' dear tell silver

Tell silver all about it

Silver keeps secrets like sand keeps sand

castles at sunsets mixed with in coming

Tide

Put a paper book in the earth and

it returns from where it came

dirt

Place me in the soil and eventually

I will reside with the rest of my lying

savage cohorts

On "The Great Pacific Garbage Patch"

Fingers to your lips

Shh, Shh, Shh

Tell no one

Tell no one that in truth I am polluting

the planet, stealing your countries

wealth and making an open

mockery of everything sacred

Yes my dear tell silver all about it.

"The silver rings are computers and

CD downloads and flash drives.

Plastic is never totally disintegrated."

(Please research the documentary

Plastic Paradise: The Great

Pacific Garbage Patch.)

"I Am a Human Embryo"

by

Regina Lee Hooper

You denied me the warmth
of my mother's womb
You turned me into a genetics
experiment.

HEK 293 Human Embryo Kidney

Human tissue to make anti-aging

facial creams , flavor soda , food and

to grow vaccines,monkey kidney too filthy?

Cannibalism?

Van Der Eb knew, Van Der Eb knows

There are millions if not billions or

trillions of us worldwide

I may never know the warmth of

a soft blanket about my body.

sweet kisses to my tiny cheeks

by brothers and sisters.

Never to hear words like "I see

Auntie's soft brown eyes there or

yes that is Daddy's smile.

We are laid bare here in cold

steel storage containers.

My potential may never be

known by this world.

There are days I cringe in horror.

Sometimes the keepers

simply press a button

And millions of us die here

in a moments breathe

I am bathed in my own tears

Will someone speak for me

My screams of former years

have gone unheeded

I am a Baby

I am a Human.

I am an Embryo.